THE BLUE ZONES DIET PROGRAM

Simple Tips for Eating and Living Like the World's Healthiest People

Janie Dolan

INTRODUCTION

Explanation Of The Blue Zone Diet Program

The Blue Zone Diet Program is a diet plan based on the dietary habits of the people who live in the Blue Zones, which are regions of the world where people are known to live longer and healthier lives. The program is based on the concept that by adopting the dietary habits of these communities, people can improve their overall health and longevity. The Blue Zone Diet Program was created by Dan Buettner, a National Geographic Fellow, who studied the dietary habits of people living in Blue Zones.

The Blue Zone Diet Program is not a strict diet plan, but rather a set of guidelines for healthy eating. The program emphasizes the consumption of plant-based foods, whole grains, legumes, and nuts, and limits the consumption of meat, processed foods, and sugary drinks. The program also encourages people to eat smaller portions and to eat slowly, as well as to avoid overeating and snacking.

One of the main principles of the Blue Zone Diet Program is the 80% rule, which suggests that people should stop eating when they are 80% full. This helps to prevent overeating, which can lead to weight gain and other health problems. Another principle of the program is the emphasis on social and family connections, as well as physical activity, as important factors in overall health and well-being.

The Blue Zone Diet Program is based on extensive research and is backed by science. Studies have shown that people who follow a plant-based diet, such as the one recommended by the Blue Zone Diet Program, are at a lower risk for chronic diseases such as heart disease, diabetes, and cancer. Additionally, people who live in Blue Zones have been found to have lower rates of these diseases, as well as lower rates of obesity and other health problems.

Overall, the Blue Zone Diet Program offers a practical and achievable way to improve overall health and longevity through simple changes in dietary habits. By adopting the principles of the program, people can enjoy the benefits of a healthier lifestyle and potentially add years to their lives.

Why It's Important To Follow A Healthy Diet

A healthy diet is essential for maintaining good health and preventing chronic diseases. The food we eat provides our bodies with the nutrients it needs to function properly, and a diet that is high in unhealthy fats, sugars, and processed foods can lead to a variety of health problems.

Eating a healthy diet can help to reduce the risk of heart disease, diabetes, and certain types of cancer. A diet that is high in fruits, vegetables, whole grains, and lean protein can provide the body with the nutrients it needs to maintain good health and prevent disease.

In addition to preventing chronic diseases, a healthy diet can also improve overall well-being. Eating a diet that is rich in nutrients can improve energy levels, mental clarity, and mood. A healthy diet can also help to maintain a healthy weight, which is important for overall health and reducing the risk of obesity-related health problems.

It's important to note that a healthy diet is not just about what you eat, but also about how much you eat. Portion control is an important aspect of a healthy diet, as overeating can lead to weight gain and other health problems.

What To Expect From The Program

The Blue Zone Diet Program offers a practical and achievable way to improve overall health and longevity through simple changes in dietary habits. By following the program, people can expect to see a variety of benefits, including:

- Improved overall health: By eating a diet that is rich in nutrients and low in unhealthy fats, sugars and processed foods, people can improve their overall health. This can include improved energy levels, better mental clarity, and a stronger immune system.

- Reduced risk of chronic diseases: The Blue Zone Diet Program is based on dietary habits that have been shown to reduce the risk of chronic diseases such as heart disease, diabetes, and certain types of cancer. By following the program, people can reduce their risk of developing these diseases and enjoy better long-term health.

- Weight loss: The Blue Zone Diet Program emphasizes portion control and the consumption of nutrient-dense foods. By following these principles, people can lose weight and maintain a healthy weight over time.

- Improved digestion: The Blue Zone Diet Program

is based on whole, unprocessed foods that are rich in fiber. By consuming these foods, people can improve their digestive health and reduce the risk of digestive problems such as constipation and bloating.

- Improved mental health: The Blue Zone Diet Program emphasizes the consumption of plant-based foods, which are rich in nutrients that are important for brain health. By following the program, people can improve their mental clarity, mood, and overall mental health.

Overall, the Blue Zone Diet Program is a comprehensive program that offers a variety of benefits for those who follow it. By adopting the principles of the program, people can improve their overall health, reduce their risk of chronic diseases, and enjoy better long-term well-being.

CHAPTER ONE

What are Blue Zones?

Explanation Of Blue Zones

Blue Zones are regions of the world where people are known to live longer, healthier lives than the rest of the world's population. The term "Blue Zone" was first coined by National Geographic Fellow and author Dan Buettner, who studied areas of high longevity across the world. Buettner identified five Blue Zones: Okinawa, Japan; Sardinia, Italy; Nicoya, Costa Rica; Ikaria, Greece; and Loma Linda, California. These regions share common characteristics that contribute to the exceptional longevity of their populations.

One of the defining characteristics of Blue Zones is their emphasis on community and social connections. The residents of Blue Zones tend to have close-knit relationships with their family and friends, which provides them with emotional support and a sense of purpose. Additionally, people in Blue Zones tend to be physically active throughout their lives, often engaging in low-intensity activities like walking, gardening, and other forms of manual labor.

Another factor contributing to the longevity of Blue Zone

populations is their diet. People in Blue Zones tend to consume a plant-based diet that is high in whole foods and low in processed foods. This means that their diets are rich in fruits, vegetables, legumes, and whole grains, which provide essential nutrients and fiber while minimizing the intake of saturated fats and added sugars.

Overall, the concept of Blue Zones provides insight into the factors that contribute to living a long and healthy life. By studying the lifestyles of people in Blue Zones, we can identify ways to improve our own health and wellbeing.

Characteristics Of Blue Zones

As mentioned earlier, Blue Zones are regions of the world where people live longer, healthier lives than the rest of the world's population. While the specific characteristics of each Blue Zone may vary slightly, there are some general traits that they share.

One key characteristic of Blue Zones is their emphasis on community and social connections. People in Blue Zones tend to have strong relationships with their family and friends, which provide them with emotional support and a sense of purpose. This social connectedness helps to reduce stress and promote a positive outlook on life.

Another characteristic of Blue Zones is their focus on physical activity. People in Blue Zones tend to engage in low-intensity physical activities throughout their lives, such as walking, gardening, and other forms of manual labor. This constant movement helps to keep their bodies healthy and fit, while also providing a sense of purpose and fulfillment.

In addition to social connections and physical activity, Blue Zones are also characterized by their diet. People in Blue Zones tend to eat a plant-based diet that is high in whole foods and low in processed foods. This means that their diets are rich in fruits, vegetables, legumes, and whole grains, which provide essential nutrients and fiber while minimizing the intake of saturated fats and added sugars.

Overall, the characteristics of Blue Zones provide insight into the lifestyle factors that contribute to living a long and healthy life. By incorporating these traits into our own lives, we can improve our health and wellbeing.

How Diet Contributes To Longevity In Blue Zones

As mentioned earlier, one of the key characteristics of Blue Zones is their focus on a plant-based diet that is high in whole foods and low in processed foods. This type of diet has been shown to have numerous health benefits that contribute to longevity.

One way in which the Blue Zone diet promotes longevity is by providing essential nutrients and fiber. Fruits, vegetables, legumes, and whole grains are all rich in vitamins, minerals, and other nutrients that are important for maintaining good health. Additionally, these foods are high in fiber, which helps to promote healthy digestion and reduce the risk of chronic diseases like heart disease and type 2 diabetes.

Another way in which the Blue Zone diet promotes longevity is by minimizing the intake of saturated fats and added sugars. These types of foods are often found in processed foods, which are not commonly consumed in

Blue Zones. Saturated fats can increase the risk of heart disease, while added sugars can lead to obesity and type 2 diabetes.

In addition to the nutrient-rich and low-fat nature of the Blue Zone diet, the way food is prepared and consumed is also important. For example, people in Blue Zones tend to eat slowly and in smaller portions, which can help with digestion and prevent overeating. Additionally, many Blue Zone cultures have traditions around food and mealtime, such as the Mediterranean tradition of gathering around a table with family and friends for a leisurely meal.

Overall, the Blue Zone diet promotes longevity by providing essential nutrients, minimizing the intake of unhealthy fats and sugars, and emphasizing a healthy approach to food and mealtime. By incorporating some of these principles into our own diets, we can improve our health and potentially live longer, healthier lives.

CHAPTER TWO

*Principles of the Blue
Zone Diet Program*

Plant-Based Eating

Plant-based eating is a way of eating that emphasizes whole, minimally processed foods from plants. This means that fruits, vegetables, legumes, nuts, and seeds are the focus of the diet, while animal products such as meat, dairy, and eggs are consumed in smaller amounts or not at all. There are several benefits associated with a plant-based diet, including improved health outcomes, environmental sustainability, and ethical considerations.

One of the main health benefits of a plant-based diet is that it is high in fiber, vitamins, and minerals, while also being low in saturated fat and cholesterol. This can lead to improved heart health, a lower risk of certain types of cancer, and better management of chronic diseases such as diabetes and high blood pressure. Plant-based diets have also been shown to be more sustainable for the environment, as they require fewer resources such as water and land to produce than animal-based diets.

To follow a plant-based diet, it's important to focus on consuming a variety of whole, minimally processed plant foods. This can include fruits and vegetables in a range of colors, whole grains such as brown rice and quinoa, legumes like lentils and chickpeas, and nuts and seeds. While animal products can still be consumed in moderation, plant-based eaters may choose to substitute them with plant-based sources of protein such as tofu, tempeh, and seitan.

Healthy Fats

Healthy fats are a crucial component of a healthy diet, as they are important for cell function, hormone production, and nutrient absorption. However, not all fats are created equal. Saturated and trans fats, which are commonly found in animal products and processed foods, can increase the risk of heart disease and other health problems. On the other hand, unsaturated fats, which are found in foods such as nuts, seeds, and avocados, can have a range of health benefits.

Monounsaturated and polyunsaturated fats are two types of unsaturated fats that are particularly beneficial for health. Monounsaturated fats can help to lower LDL (bad) cholesterol levels and reduce the risk of heart disease, while polyunsaturated fats are essential fatty acids that the body cannot produce on its own. Omega-3 fatty acids, which are a type of polyunsaturated fat, have been shown to reduce inflammation and improve brain function.

To increase your intake of healthy fats, try incorporating foods such as nuts, seeds, avocados, and fatty fish like salmon into your diet. It's important to consume these foods in moderation, as they are still high in calories. It's also important to limit your intake of saturated and trans fats by choosing leaner cuts of meat, opting for low-fat dairy products, and avoiding processed foods.

Lean Proteins

Protein is an essential macronutrient that is important for building and repairing tissues in the body. However, not all sources of protein are created equal. While animal products such as meat, eggs, and dairy are high in protein, they can also be high in saturated fat and cholesterol. Plant-based sources of protein, on the other hand, are generally lower in fat and can also provide additional nutrients such as fiber and antioxidants.

To increase your intake of lean proteins, consider incorporating more plant-based sources of protein into your diet. This can include legumes such as lentils and chickpeas, tofu and other soy products, nuts and seeds, and whole grains such as quinoa and brown rice. Animal-based sources of protein can still be consumed in moderation, but it's important to choose leaner cuts of meat and avoid processed meats such as bacon and sausage.

In addition to being a source of protein, plant-based proteins can also provide additional health benefits. For example, legumes are high in fiber and can help to reduce cholesterol levels, while nuts and seeds are rich in healthy fats and can help to lower inflammation in the body. By choosing a variety of lean protein sources, you can ensure that you are getting all the nutrients your body needs to function at its best.

Whole Grains

Whole grains are an important part of a healthy diet, as they are rich in fiber, vitamins, and minerals. Unlike refined grains, which have had the bran and germ removed during processing, whole grains contain all parts of the grain, providing additional nutrients and health benefits. Whole grains have been linked to a reduced risk of heart disease, diabetes, and certain types of cancer.

Examples of whole grains include brown rice, quinoa, whole wheat, barley, and oats. These grains can be incorporated into a variety of dishes, from salads to soups to breakfast porridge. When choosing whole grain products, it's important to read labels carefully, as many products are marketed as "whole grain" but still contain a significant amount of refined grains.

To increase your intake of whole grains, try substituting white rice or pasta with brown rice or whole wheat pasta, or choose whole grain breads and cereals. By incorporating more whole grains into your diet, you can improve your health and reduce the risk of chronic diseases.

Low Sugar Intake

Excess sugar intake has been linked to a range of health problems, including obesity, type 2 diabetes, and heart disease. While some amount of sugar is necessary for energy and brain function, it's important to limit your intake of added sugars, which are commonly found in processed foods such as candy, soda, and baked goods.

To reduce your sugar intake, try to limit your consumption of processed foods and focus on whole, minimally processed foods instead. This can include fruits, vegetables, whole grains, and lean protein sources. When choosing packaged foods, read labels carefully and look for products with little to no added sugars.

It's also important to be aware of hidden sources of sugar, such as in condiments like ketchup and barbecue sauce, or in beverages such as fruit juice and sports drinks. By reducing your intake of added sugars and focusing on whole, nutrient-dense foods, you can improve your health and reduce the risk of chronic diseases.

Intermittent Fasting

Intermittent fasting is a dietary approach that involves cycling between periods of fasting and periods of eating. While there are several different approaches to intermittent fasting, the most common method involves limiting food intake to an eight-hour window each day, and fasting for the remaining 16 hours.

Intermittent fasting has been linked to a range of health benefits, including weight loss, improved insulin sensitivity, and reduced inflammation. It has also been shown to be a safe and effective approach for weight loss and improving overall health.

To try intermittent fasting, start by gradually increasing the amount of time you fast each day. For example, you may start by fasting for 12 hours overnight, and gradually increase to 14 or 16 hours over time. It's important to ensure that you are still consuming enough calories and nutrients during your eating window, and to speak with a healthcare professional before starting any new dietary approach.

In conclusion, plant-based eating, healthy fats, lean

proteins, whole grains, low sugar intake, and intermittent fasting are all dietary approaches that can have a range of health benefits. By incorporating these approaches into your diet and lifestyle, you can improve your health, reduce the risk of chronic diseases, and feel your best.

CHAPTER THREE

Increased Lifespan

One of the most significant benefits of advancements in medical science and technology is the increased lifespan of human beings. Life expectancy has been on the rise over the past few decades, and the trend is likely to continue in the coming years. According to the World Health Organization (WHO), global life expectancy has increased from 64.2 years in 1990 to 72.6 years in 2019. This increase in lifespan has several implications for individuals and society as a whole.

As people age, they are more likely to suffer from chronic diseases, such as diabetes, heart disease, and cancer. However, with advances in medical science, people can now live longer while managing these chronic conditions more effectively. For instance, new treatments and medications can help people with diabetes to manage their blood sugar levels and reduce their risk of complications.

This trend has significant implications for healthcare systems and social services, as older adults are more likely to require medical care and social support. In response, governments and healthcare providers must adapt to the changing needs of an aging population, by investing in new technologies, services, and policies that cater to the needs of older adults.

Increased lifespan also has economic implications for individuals and society. People who live longer can continue to work and contribute to the economy for a more extended period, which can have positive effects on economic growth and productivity. Additionally, older adults who remain healthy and active can participate in social and cultural activities, which can contribute to a more vibrant and diverse society.

However, it is important to note that increased lifespan is not without its challenges. As people live longer, they may require more healthcare and social support, which can put a strain on healthcare systems and social services. Additionally, older adults may face new challenges related to social isolation, ageism, and age-related discrimination, which can impact their quality of life.

Overall, increased lifespan is a significant achievement of modern medicine and technology, with important implications for individuals and society as a whole. While there are challenges associated with an aging population, there are also opportunities for innovation and growth, as people continue to live longer and healthier lives.

Lower Risk Of Chronic Diseases

Chronic diseases, such as heart disease, stroke, cancer, and diabetes, are a leading cause of death and disability worldwide. However, advances in medical science and technology have led to new treatments and preventative measures that can lower the risk of chronic diseases. These measures have important implications for public health and individual wellbeing.

One of the most effective ways to lower the risk of chronic diseases is through lifestyle changes. A healthy diet, regular exercise, and avoiding tobacco and excessive alcohol consumption can all lower the risk of chronic diseases. Additionally, early detection and treatment of chronic diseases can prevent complications and improve outcomes. For instance, regular screenings for cancer can detect the disease at an early stage, when it is more treatable.

New treatments and medications are also available to lower the risk of chronic diseases. For example, statins are drugs that can lower cholesterol levels and reduce the risk of heart disease. Similarly, new immunotherapies are being developed that can boost the immune system and target cancer cells. These treatments can improve outcomes and quality of life for people with chronic diseases.

Preventative measures, such as vaccinations, can also lower the risk of chronic diseases. For instance, vaccinations against the human papillomavirus (HPV) can prevent cervical cancer, while vaccines against the flu can prevent complications in people with chronic conditions.

Lowering the risk of chronic diseases has important implications for public health and individual wellbeing. Chronic diseases are often expensive to treat and can significantly impact an individual's quality of life. By lowering the risk of these diseases, people can live healthier and more productive lives, which can have positive effects on society as a whole.

However, there are still challenges associated with preventing and treating chronic diseases. For instance, access to healthcare and preventative measures can be limited in some communities, which can disproportionately impact marginalized populations. Additionally, there is still much to learn about the causes and risk factors of chronic diseases, which can make prevention and treatment more challenging.

Despite these challenges, the increasing availability of preventative measures, treatments, and lifestyle changes that can lower the risk of chronic diseases is a significant achievement of modern medicine and technology. By continuing to invest in research and development, healthcare systems can continue to improve outcomes for people with chronic conditions, and prevent these diseases from becoming a significant public health burden.

Improved Mental Health

Mental health is an essential component of overall wellbeing, and advances in medical science and technology have led to new treatments and preventative measures that can improve mental health outcomes. Mental health conditions, such as depression, anxiety, and post-traumatic stress disorder (PTSD), are prevalent and can have significant impacts on individuals and society as a whole.

One of the most significant developments in mental health treatment has been the introduction of new medications and therapies. Antidepressants and anti-anxiety medications, for instance, can help manage symptoms of depression and anxiety, and improve overall quality of life. Additionally, new therapies, such as cognitive-behavioral therapy (CBT) and mindfulness-based therapy, can help individuals learn coping strategies and manage their mental health conditions more effectively.

Improved access to mental healthcare is also critical in improving mental health outcomes. With telehealth and virtual therapy, individuals can access mental health services from the comfort of their own homes, which can reduce barriers to care and improve outcomes. Additionally, increased funding for mental healthcare and greater integration of mental healthcare into primary care can ensure that individuals with mental health conditions receive the care and support they need.

Preventative measures, such as mental health education and public awareness campaigns, can also improve mental health outcomes. By reducing stigma and increasing awareness about mental health conditions, individuals may be more likely to seek care and support, which can prevent mental health conditions from becoming more severe.

While there are still challenges associated with improving mental health outcomes, such as limited access to care and resources, the increasing availability of effective treatments, improved access to care, and preventative measures is a significant achievement of modern medicine and technology. By continuing to invest in research and development, healthcare systems can continue to improve mental health outcomes and reduce the burden of mental health conditions on individuals and society as a whole.

Increased Energy And Vitality

Feeling energetic and vital is essential for overall wellbeing, and advances in medical science and technology have led to new treatments and preventative measures that can improve energy levels and vitality. Fatigue and decreased energy levels are common symptoms of many medical conditions, such as chronic fatigue syndrome and fibromyalgia, and can significantly impact an individual's quality of life.

One of the most effective ways to improve energy levels and vitality is through lifestyle changes. Regular exercise, a healthy diet, and stress management techniques, such as meditation and yoga, can all improve energy levels and reduce fatigue. Additionally, addressing underlying medical conditions, such as anemia or thyroid disorders, can improve energy levels and vitality.

New treatments and medications are also available to improve energy levels and vitality. For instance, medications for chronic fatigue syndrome, such as modafinil, can improve energy levels and reduce fatigue. Additionally, new therapies, such as transcranial magnetic stimulation (TMS), can stimulate brain activity and improve energy levels in individuals with depression or other mental health conditions.

Improved sleep hygiene can also improve energy levels and vitality. Sleep disorders, such as sleep apnea, can cause fatigue and decrease energy levels. By addressing these disorders through treatments such as continuous positive airway pressure (CPAP) machines, individuals can experience improved sleep and increased energy levels.

While there are still challenges associated with improving energy levels and vitality, such as addressing underlying medical conditions and improving sleep hygiene, the increasing availability of effective treatments and lifestyle changes is a significant achievement of modern medicine and technology. By continuing to invest in research and development, healthcare systems can continue to improve energy levels and vitality, which can have positive effects on individuals and society as a whole.

In conclusion, advances in medical science and technology have led to numerous achievements in improving public health and individual wellbeing. Increased lifespan, lower risk of chronic diseases, improved mental health, and increased energy and vitality are all significant accomplishments that have resulted from research and development in healthcare. While challenges still exist, continued investment in research and development can lead to even more significant achievements in the future, and improve outcomes for individuals and society as a whole.

CHAPTER FOUR

*Getting Started on the Blue
Zone Diet Program*

Steps To Take Before Starting The Program

Before starting a new program, it is important to take certain steps to ensure that you are setting yourself up for success. These steps can help you prepare both mentally and physically for the changes that will come with the program. Here are some key steps to take before starting a new program:

1. Define your goals: Take some time to think about what you hope to achieve through the program. Write down your goals and be specific. Do you want to lose weight? Build muscle? Improve your endurance? Having clear goals will help you stay focused and motivated.

2. Assess your current fitness level: Before starting a new program, it is important to assess your current fitness level. This will help you determine where you are starting from and track your progress as you go. You can assess your fitness level by measuring your body composition, cardiovascular endurance, muscular strength, and flexibility.

3. Consult with a healthcare professional: Before starting any new program, it is important to consult with a healthcare professional. This can be your primary care physician, a registered dietitian, or a certified personal trainer. They can help you determine if the program is safe and appropriate for you, given any medical conditions or injuries you may have.

4. Set a realistic timeline: It is important to set a realistic timeline for achieving your goals. This will help you stay motivated and avoid frustration. Be sure to take into account any upcoming events or vacations that may impact your progress.

5. Plan your workouts and meals: Before starting the program, plan your workouts and meals in advance. This will help you stay on track and avoid making impulsive decisions. Consider scheduling your workouts and meal prep time in your calendar to make them a priority.

Taking these steps before starting a program can help you set yourself up for success and achieve your goals. Remember, it is important to be patient and consistent in your efforts. Results may not come overnight, but with time and effort, you will see progress.

Meal Planning And Preparation

Meal planning and preparation is an essential component of any successful nutrition program. It can help you stay on track with your dietary goals, save time and money, and reduce stress. Here are some tips for effective meal planning and preparation:

1. Set aside time for planning: Set aside a specific time each week to plan your meals for the upcoming week. Consider your schedule for the week ahead and plan meals that are easy to prepare and fit into your busy schedule.

2. Make a grocery list: Once you have planned your meals, make a grocery list of all the ingredients you will need. This can help you avoid making impulsive purchases and stick to your budget.

3. Prep ingredients in advance: Spend some time each week prepping ingredients in advance. Chop vegetables, cook grains and proteins, and store them in containers in the fridge or freezer. This can help you save time when it comes to preparing meals during the week.

4. Batch cook: Consider batch cooking meals that can be easily reheated throughout the week. This can save you time and ensure that you always have healthy meals on hand.

5. Invest in quality storage containers: Invest in high-quality storage containers that are easy to clean and can be used in the fridge, freezer, and microwave. This can help you store and reheat meals safely and efficiently.

6. Get creative: Don't be afraid to get creative with your meal planning and preparation. Experiment with new ingredients and recipes to keep things interesting and prevent boredom.

By incorporating these tips into your meal planning and preparation routine, you can make healthy eating easier and more enjoyable.

Tips For Dining Out And Socializing

Dining out and socializing can be challenging when trying to stick to a nutrition program.

However, with a little planning and preparation, it is possible to enjoy social events while still staying on track with your goals. Here are some tips for dining out and socializing:

1. Research the menu: Before going out to eat, research the restaurant's menu online. Look for healthy options that fit within your dietary goals. Most restaurants will have nutrition information available upon request.

2. Make special requests: Don't be afraid to make special requests when ordering. Ask for dressings or sauces on the side, substitute vegetables for starchy sides, or ask for grilled or baked options instead of fried.

3. Control portions: Many restaurants serve large portions, which can make it difficult to stick to your dietary goals. Consider sharing a meal with a friend or taking half of your meal home for later.

4. Stay hydrated: Drink plenty of water throughout the meal to help you feel full and avoid overeating. Avoid sugary drinks and alcohol, which can add empty calories.

5. Plan ahead for social events: If you know you will be attending a social event where food will be served, plan ahead. Eat a healthy snack beforehand so you are not overly hungry when you arrive. Bring a healthy dish to share, or offer to host the event so you can control the menu.

By following these tips, you can enjoy dining out and socializing while still staying on track with your dietary goals.

Overcoming Common Challenges

Sticking to a nutrition program can be challenging,

especially in the face of common obstacles such as cravings, busy schedules, and social pressures. Here are some tips for overcoming common challenges:

1. Manage cravings: Cravings for unhealthy foods can be a major obstacle to sticking to a nutrition program. To manage cravings, try drinking water, distracting yourself with a healthy activity, or substituting a healthier option.

2. Plan ahead: Busy schedules can make it difficult to stick to a nutrition program. To stay on track, plan your meals and workouts in advance. Use a meal planning app or calendar to help you stay organized.

3. Find support: Social support can be a powerful motivator when it comes to sticking to a nutrition program. Find a workout buddy or join a support group to help you stay on track and stay motivated.

4. Practice mindfulness: Mindfulness can help you stay present and focused on your goals. Take time to slow down and savor your meals, and practice mindful breathing or meditation to manage stress and anxiety.

5. Focus on progress, not perfection: Remember that progress, not perfection, is the key to success. Don't beat yourself up if you slip up or make a mistake. Instead, focus on the progress you have made and the small steps you can take to continue moving forward.

By following these tips, you can overcome common challenges and stick to your nutrition program, achieving your goals and improving your overall health and well-being.

CHAPTER FIVE.

*Recipes for the Blue
Zone Diet Program*

Breakfast

Oatmeal with Blueberries, Chopped Nuts, and a Drizzle of Honey

This oatmeal bowl is a hearty and nutritious breakfast option that is easy to make and customizable to suit your taste buds. The sweet blueberries, crunchy chopped nuts, and drizzle of honey make it a delicious and satisfying morning meal.

Ingredients:

- 1 cup rolled oats
- 2 cups water
- 1/4 teaspoon salt
- 1/2 cup blueberries
- 1/4 cup chopped nuts (such as almonds or walnuts)
- 1 tablespoon honey

Instructions:

1. In a medium-sized saucepan, bring the oats,

water, and salt to a boil over high heat.

2. Reduce the heat to low and simmer for 5-10 minutes, stirring occasionally, until the oats are cooked and the mixture has thickened to your desired consistency.

3. Divide the oatmeal into two bowls.

4. Top each bowl with blueberries, chopped nuts, and a drizzle of honey.

5. Serve immediately.

Nutritional Information:

- Calories: 377
- Protein: 10g
- Fat: 11g
- Carbohydrates: 63g
- Fiber: 8g

Vegetable and Egg Scramble with Spinach, Onions, and Bell Peppers

This vegetable and egg scramble is a tasty and healthy breakfast that is packed with protein and vegetables. It's a great way to start your day and provides you with energy to get through the morning.

Ingredients:

- 2 tablespoons olive oil
- 1/2 onion, diced
- 1/2 bell pepper, diced
- 2 cups spinach
- 4 eggs
- Salt and pepper, to taste

Instructions:

1. Heat the olive oil in a non-stick pan over medium heat.

2. Add the onions and bell peppers and sauté for 2-3 minutes until they are slightly softened.

3. Add the spinach to the pan and sauté until wilted.

4. In a separate bowl, beat the eggs together with salt and pepper to taste.

5. Pour the eggs over the vegetables and stir gently until the eggs are cooked to your desired consistency.

6. Serve immediately.

Nutritional Information:

- Calories: 282
- Protein: 16g
- Fat: 22g
- Carbohydrates: 8g
- Fiber: 2g

Whole Grain Toast Topped with Avocado, Tomato, and a Poached Egg

This breakfast option is a delicious and healthy way to start your day. It provides a balanced combination of healthy fats, protein, and complex carbohydrates to keep you full and satisfied throughout the morning.

Ingredients:

- 2 slices whole grain bread, toasted
- 1/2 avocado, sliced
- 1/2 tomato, sliced

- 1 poached egg
- Salt and pepper, to taste

Instructions:

1. Toast the whole grain bread to your desired level of doneness.
2. Slice the avocado and tomato and arrange them on top of the toast.
3. Poach the egg to your desired level of doneness.
4. Place the poached egg on top of the avocado and tomato.
5. Season with salt and pepper to taste.
6. Serve immediately.

Nutritional Information:

- Calories: 348
- Protein: 17g
- Fat: 20g
- Carbohydrates: 29g
- Fiber: 10g

Greek Yogurt with Sliced Banana, Almonds, and a Sprinkle of Cinnamon

This Greek yogurt bowl is a simple and delicious breakfast option that is easy to prepare and full of nutrients. The combination of creamy yogurt, sweet banana, crunchy almonds, and warm cinnamon make it a flavorful and satisfying meal.

Ingredients:

- 1 cup Greek yogurt
- 1 banana, sliced

- 1/4 cup sliced almonds
- 1/4 teaspoon cinnamon

Instructions:

1. In a bowl, add the Greek yogurt and spread it out evenly.

2. Add the sliced banana on top of the yogurt.

3. Sprinkle the sliced almonds and cinnamon over the top of the banana and yogurt.

4. Serve immediately.

Nutritional Information:

- Calories: 354
- Protein: 24g
- Fat: 14g
- Carbohydrates: 37g
- Fiber: 6g

Quinoa Breakfast Bowl with Roasted Sweet Potatoes, Black Beans, and Salsa

This quinoa breakfast bowl is a protein-packed and satisfying meal that will keep you full throughout the morning. The combination of sweet potatoes, black beans, and salsa make it a flavorful and nutritious breakfast option.

Ingredients:

- 1 cup cooked quinoa
- 1 medium sweet potato, peeled and cubed
- 1/2 can black beans, rinsed and drained
- 1/4 cup salsa

Instructions:

1. Preheat the oven to 400°F (200°C).

2. Place the cubed sweet potato on a baking sheet and drizzle with olive oil.

3. Roast the sweet potato in the oven for 20-25 minutes, or until they are tender and golden brown.

4. In a bowl, add the cooked quinoa, roasted sweet potato, and black beans.

5. Top with salsa and mix well.

6. Serve immediately.

Nutritional Information:

- Calories: 386
- Protein: 14g
- Fat: 3g
- Carbohydrates: 78g
- Fiber: 15g

Smoothie Bowl Made with Frozen Berries, Almond Milk, Spinach, and a Scoop of Protein Powder, Topped with Granola and Sliced Banana

This smoothie bowl is a nutritious and refreshing breakfast option that is easy to make and customize to your taste. The combination of frozen berries, spinach, and protein powder make it a great way to start your day.

Ingredients:

- 1 cup frozen mixed berries
- 1/2 cup almond milk
- 1 cup spinach

- 1 scoop protein powder
- 1/4 cup granola
- 1 banana, sliced

Instructions:

1. In a blender, add the frozen mixed berries, almond milk, spinach, and protein powder.

2. Blend until the mixture is smooth and creamy.

3. Pour the smoothie into a bowl.

4. Top the smoothie with granola and sliced banana.

5. Serve immediately.

Nutritional Information:

- Calories: 453
- Protein: 30g
- Fat: 11g
- Carbohydrates: 66g
- Fiber: 13g

Whole Grain Toast Topped with Avocado, Tomato, and a Poached Egg

This savory and satisfying breakfast option is full of healthy fats, fiber, and protein. The combination of creamy avocado, juicy tomato, and runny poached egg make it a delicious and filling meal.

Ingredients:

- 2 slices whole grain bread, toasted
- 1 avocado, mashed
- 1 tomato, sliced
- 2 eggs

- Salt and pepper, to taste

Instructions:

1. Toast the whole grain bread until it is lightly browned.

2. Spread the mashed avocado on top of each slice of bread.

3. Add the sliced tomato on top of the avocado.

4. Poach the eggs in a pot of boiling water until the whites are set but the yolks are still runny.

5. Place one poached egg on top of each slice of toast.

6. Sprinkle with salt and pepper to taste.

7. Serve immediately.

Nutritional Information:

- Calories: 433
- Protein: 20g
- Fat: 25g
- Carbohydrates: 35g
- Fiber: 13g

Lunch

Quinoa Salad with Grilled Vegetables

This Quinoa Salad with Grilled Vegetables is a perfect meal for a warm summer day. It is packed with nutritious ingredients that will leave you feeling satisfied and energized. The dish is a colorful combination of quinoa, grilled vegetables, and a zesty lemon dressing.

Ingredients:

- 1 cup quinoa
- 2 cups water
- 1 red pepper, sliced
- 1 zucchini, sliced
- 1 yellow squash, sliced
- 1 red onion, sliced
- 2 tbsp. olive oil
- Salt and pepper
- 1 tbsp. fresh parsley, chopped
- 1/4 cup feta cheese, crumbled

For the dressing:

- 1/4 cup olive oil
- 2 tbsp. lemon juice
- 1 tbsp. Dijon mustard
- 1 tbsp. honey
- Salt and pepper

Instructions:

1. Rinse the quinoa and put it in a pot with 2 cups of water. Bring it to a boil, then reduce the heat and let it simmer for 15-20 minutes, until the water is absorbed.

2. While the quinoa is cooking, prepare the vegetables. Brush them with olive oil and sprinkle with salt and pepper.

3. Heat a grill pan or grill to medium-high heat. Grill the vegetables until they are lightly charred, about 3-4 minutes per side.

4. In a small bowl, whisk together the olive oil,

lemon juice, Dijon mustard, honey, salt, and pepper.

5. In a large bowl, mix together the cooked quinoa, grilled vegetables, and chopped parsley. Pour the dressing over the salad and toss to combine.

6. Sprinkle crumbled feta cheese over the top of the salad.

Nutritional information:

This Quinoa Salad with Grilled Vegetables serves 4. Each serving contains approximately:

- Calories: 355
- Fat: 23g
- Protein: 7g
- Carbohydrates: 31g
- Fiber: 5g
- Sugar: 8g

Lentil Soup with Fresh Vegetables

This Lentil Soup with Fresh Vegetables is a hearty and healthy meal that is perfect for a cozy night in. The soup is filled with protein-rich lentils and fresh vegetables, making it a nutritious and satisfying dish.

Ingredients:

- 2 cups brown lentils
- 1 onion, chopped
- 3 cloves garlic, minced
- 2 carrots, chopped
- 2 celery stalks, chopped
- 1 tbsp. olive oil

- 1 tsp. ground cumin
- 1/2 tsp. ground coriander
- 6 cups vegetable broth
- 1 cup fresh spinach
- Salt and pepper

Instructions:

1. Rinse the lentils and soak them in water for at least 1 hour.

2. In a large pot, heat the olive oil over medium heat. Add the onion and garlic and cook until the onion is translucent.

3. Add the carrots and celery and cook for 5-7 minutes, until they begin to soften.

4. Drain the lentils and add them to the pot with the vegetables. Add the cumin and coriander and stir to combine.

5. Pour in the vegetable broth and bring the soup to a boil. Reduce the heat and let the soup simmer for 30-40 minutes, until the lentils are tender.

6. Add the fresh spinach to the pot and stir until it is wilted. Season with salt and pepper to taste.

Nutritional information:

This Lentil Soup with Fresh Vegetables serves 6. Each serving contains approximately:

- Calories: 215
- Fat: 3g
- Protein: 14g
- Carbohydrates: 36g

- Fiber: 15g
- Sugar: 5g

Brown Rice and Tofu Stir Fry

This Brown Rice and Tofu Stir Fry is a delicious and healthy vegetarian meal. It is made with brown rice, tofu, and a variety of colorful vegetables, making it a nutrient-dense dish.

Ingredients:

- 1 cup brown rice
- 2 cups water
- 1 tbsp. olive oil
- 1 block tofu, cubed
- 1 red bell pepper, sliced
- 1 yellow bell pepper, sliced
- 1 cup snow peas
- 2 garlic cloves, minced
- 1 tsp. ginger, minced
- 2 tbsp. soy sauce
- 1 tbsp. honey
- 1 tbsp. cornstarch
- 1/4 cup vegetable broth
- Salt and pepper
- Green onions, sliced (optional)

Instructions:

1. Rinse the brown rice and put it in a pot with 2 cups of water. Bring it to a boil, then reduce the heat and let it simmer for 40-50 minutes, until the water is absorbed and the rice is tender.

2. In a large skillet or wok, heat the olive oil over medium-high heat. Add the cubed tofu and cook until lightly browned, about 5-7 minutes.

3. Add the sliced bell peppers, snow peas, minced garlic, and minced ginger to the skillet. Cook for 5-7 minutes, until the vegetables are tender.

4. In a small bowl, whisk together the soy sauce, honey, cornstarch, and vegetable broth.

5. Pour the sauce over the vegetables and tofu in the skillet. Stir until the sauce thickens and coats the vegetables and tofu.

6. Serve the stir fry over the cooked brown rice. Top with sliced green onions, if desired.

Nutritional information:

This Brown Rice and Tofu Stir Fry serves 4. Each serving contains approximately:

- Calories: 364
- Fat: 11g
- Protein: 15g
- Carbohydrates: 55g
- Fiber: 5g
- Sugar: 9g

Chickpea and Spinach Stew

This Chickpea and Spinach Stew is a vegan meal that is packed with protein, fiber, and nutrients. It is a flavorful and hearty dish that can be served over rice or with crusty bread.

Ingredients:

- 1 onion, chopped

- 3 cloves garlic, minced
- 2 cans chickpeas, drained and rinsed
- 1 can diced tomatoes
- 4 cups fresh spinach
- 1 tsp. ground cumin
- 1 tsp. paprika
- 1/4 tsp. cayenne pepper
- 2 cups vegetable broth
- Salt and pepper
- Fresh parsley, chopped (optional)

Instructions:

1. In a large pot, sauté the chopped onion and minced garlic in a bit of olive oil over medium heat until the onion is translucent.

2. Add the chickpeas, diced tomatoes, cumin, paprika, and cayenne pepper to the pot. Stir until the chickpeas are coated in the spices.

3. Pour in the vegetable broth and bring the stew to a boil. Reduce the heat and let it simmer for 20-30 minutes, until the stew thickens.

4. Stir in the fresh spinach and cook until wilted, about 3-5 minutes.

5. Season the stew with salt and pepper to taste.

6. Serve the Chickpea and Spinach Stew hot, garnished with fresh parsley if desired.

Nutritional information:

This Chickpea and Spinach Stew serves 4. Each serving contains approximately:

- Calories: 205
- Fat: 2g
- Protein: 10g
- Carbohydrates: 39g
- Fiber: 11g
- Sugar: 7g

Grilled Salmon with Roasted Sweet Potatoes

This Grilled Salmon with Roasted Sweet Potatoes is a perfect healthy dinner for seafood lovers. It is a flavorful and nutritious meal that is packed with omega-3 fatty acids and vitamins.

Ingredients:

- 4 salmon fillets, skin removed
- 1 tbsp. olive oil
- Salt and pepper
- 2 large sweet potatoes, peeled and cubed
- 1 tbsp. honey
- 1 tbsp. Dijon mustard
- 1 tbsp. apple cider vinegar
- 1 tbsp. olive oil
- Salt and pepper
- Fresh parsley, chopped (optional)

Instructions:

1. Preheat the oven to 400°F (200°C).

2. Toss the cubed sweet potatoes in 1 tablespoon of olive oil and season with salt and pepper. Place them on a baking sheet and roast for 25-30 minutes, until tender and lightly browned.

3. In a small bowl, whisk together the honey, Dijon mustard, apple cider vinegar, and 1 tablespoon of olive oil.

4. Season the salmon fillets with salt and pepper. Brush the honey mustard sauce over the fillets.

5. Preheat a grill or grill pan over medium-high heat. Grill the salmon fillets for 3-4 minutes per side, until the fish is cooked through and lightly charred.

6. Serve the grilled salmon with the roasted sweet potatoes. Garnish with chopped fresh parsley if desired.

Nutritional information:

This Grilled Salmon with Roasted Sweet Potatoes serves 4. Each serving contains approximately:

- Calories: 354
- Fat: 16g
- Protein: 27g
- Carbohydrates: 28g
- Fiber: 4g
- Sugar: 10g

Greek Salad with Grilled Chicken

This Greek Salad with Grilled Chicken is a fresh and flavorful meal that is perfect for summer. It is made with a variety of colorful vegetables, feta cheese, and grilled chicken, making it a nutrient-dense and protein-packed dish.

Ingredients:

- 2 boneless, skinless chicken breasts

- 1 tbsp. olive oil
- 1 tsp. dried oregano
- Salt and pepper
- 1 head romaine lettuce, chopped
- 1 cucumber, sliced
- 1 red onion, sliced
- 1 pint cherry tomatoes, halved
- 1/2 cup kalamata olives, pitted
- 4 oz. feta cheese, crumbled
- 1/4 cup red wine vinegar
- 1/4 cup olive oil
- 1 tsp. Dijon mustard
- 1 garlic clove, minced
- Salt and pepper

Instructions:

1. Preheat a grill or grill pan over medium-high heat.

2. Season the chicken breasts with 1 tablespoon of olive oil, dried oregano, salt, and pepper.

3. Grill the chicken breasts for 5-6 minutes per side, until they are cooked through and have grill marks.

4. Let the chicken rest for 5 minutes, then slice it.

5. In a large salad bowl, combine the chopped romaine lettuce, sliced cucumber, sliced red onion, halved cherry tomatoes, and pitted kalamata olives. Add the sliced chicken and crumbled feta cheese.

6. In a small bowl, whisk together the red wine

    vinegar, olive oil, Dijon mustard, minced garlic, salt, and pepper to make the salad dressing.

7. Drizzle the salad dressing over the Greek salad and toss to combine.

8. Serve the Greek Salad with Grilled Chicken immediately.

Nutritional information:

This Greek Salad with Grilled Chicken serves 4. Each serving contains approximately:

- Calories: 385
- Fat: 26g
- Protein: 25g
- Carbohydrates: 14g
- Fiber: 4g
- Sugar: 7g

All of these recipes are delicious, healthy, and easy to make. Whether you're a vegetarian or a seafood lover, there's something for everyone on this list. Enjoy!

Dinner

Grilled Fish with Lemon and Herbs

This grilled fish dish is a perfect healthy option for a light dinner. The lemon and herbs add a refreshing flavor to the dish, making it a great option for summer nights.

Ingredients:

- 4 fish fillets (such as salmon, sea bass, or tilapia)
- 2 lemons, juiced
- 2 tablespoons olive oil

- 2 tablespoons chopped fresh herbs (such as parsley, thyme, or dill)
- Salt and pepper to taste

Instructions:

1. Preheat grill to medium-high heat.

2. In a small bowl, whisk together the lemon juice, olive oil, chopped herbs, salt, and pepper.

3. Brush the fish fillets with the herb mixture and let sit for 5-10 minutes.

4. Grill the fish for 5-7 minutes on each side or until cooked through.

5. Serve with a side of your choice.

Nutritional Information:

- Calories: 230
- Protein: 30g
- Fat: 11g
- Carbohydrates: 2g
- Fiber: 0g

Lentil and Vegetable Stew

This lentil and vegetable stew is a hearty and satisfying meal that is packed with nutrients. The combination of lentils and vegetables makes this dish a great source of protein, fiber, vitamins, and minerals.

Ingredients:

- 1 cup dried lentils, rinsed and drained
- 4 cups vegetable broth
- 2 tablespoons olive oil
- 1 onion, chopped

- 2 garlic cloves, minced
- 2 carrots, chopped
- 2 celery stalks, chopped
- 1 sweet potato, peeled and chopped
- 1 teaspoon dried thyme
- Salt and pepper to taste

Instructions:

1. In a large pot, heat the olive oil over medium-high heat.
2. Add the onion and garlic and cook for 2-3 minutes or until softened.
3. Add the carrots, celery, and sweet potato and cook for an additional 5 minutes.
4. Add the lentils, vegetable broth, thyme, salt, and pepper and bring to a boil.
5. Reduce the heat to low and simmer for 30-40 minutes or until the lentils are tender.
6. Serve hot with a slice of bread.

Nutritional Information:

- Calories: 320
- Protein: 15g
- Fat: 7g
- Carbohydrates: 50g
- Fiber: 15g

Moroccan-style Vegetable Tagine

This Moroccan-style vegetable tagine is a flavorful and aromatic dish that is perfect for a cozy dinner at home. The combination of spices, vegetables, and chickpeas creates a delicious and hearty meal.

Ingredients:

- 2 tablespoons olive oil
- 1 onion, chopped
- 2 garlic cloves, minced
- 2 carrots, chopped
- 2 zucchinis, chopped
- 1 sweet potato, peeled and chopped
- 1 can chickpeas, drained and rinsed
- 1 teaspoon ground cumin
- 1 teaspoon ground coriander
- 1 teaspoon ground cinnamon
- 1 teaspoon paprika
- Salt and pepper to taste
- 2 cups vegetable broth
- 1/4 cup chopped fresh cilantro

Instructions:

1. In a large pot, heat the olive oil over medium-high heat.

2. Add the onion and garlic and cook for 2-3 minutes or until softened.

3. Add the carrots, zucchinis, and sweet potato and cook for an additional 5 minutes.

4. Add the chickpeas, cumin, coriander, cinnamon, paprika, salt, and pepper and stir to combine.

5. Pour the vegetable broth over the vegetables and chickpeas.

6. Bring the mixture to a boil, then reduce the heat

to low and simmer for 20-30 minutes or until the vegetables are tender and the flavors have melded together.

7. Serve hot, garnished with chopped cilantro.

Nutritional Information:

- Calories: 240
- Protein: 8g
- Fat: 6g
- Carbohydrates: 42g
- Fiber: 12g

Tofu and Vegetable Stir-Fry

This tofu and vegetable stir-fry is a quick and easy meal that is perfect for a busy weeknight. It is loaded with vegetables and tofu, making it a great source of protein and nutrients.

Ingredients:

- 1 block tofu, drained and cubed
- 2 tablespoons soy sauce
- 1 tablespoon cornstarch
- 1 tablespoon vegetable oil
- 1 onion, chopped
- 2 garlic cloves, minced
- 2 cups mixed vegetables (such as broccoli, carrots, and bell peppers)
- 1/4 cup vegetable broth
- Salt and pepper to taste

Instructions:

1. In a small bowl, whisk together the soy sauce and

cornstarch.

2. Heat the vegetable oil in a large skillet or wok over medium-high heat.

3. Add the tofu and cook for 5-7 minutes or until browned on all sides.

4. Remove the tofu from the skillet and set aside.

5. Add the onion and garlic to the skillet and cook for 2-3 minutes or until softened.

6. Add the mixed vegetables and cook for an additional 5 minutes or until tender.

7. Pour the vegetable broth over the vegetables and stir in the soy sauce mixture.

8. Add the tofu back to the skillet and stir to combine.

9. Cook for an additional 2-3 minutes or until the sauce has thickened and everything is heated through.

10. Serve hot over rice or noodles.

Nutritional Information:

- Calories: 250
- Protein: 15g
- Fat: 10g
- Carbohydrates: 25g
- Fiber: 6g

Quinoa and Roasted Vegetable Salad with Balsamic Vinaigrette

This quinoa and roasted vegetable salad is a delicious and healthy option for lunch or dinner. The combination of quinoa, roasted vegetables, and balsamic vinaigrette creates a flavorful and filling meal.

Ingredients:

- 1 cup quinoa, rinsed and drained
- 2 cups water
- 2 tablespoons olive oil
- 2 cups mixed vegetables (such as bell peppers, zucchini, and cherry tomatoes)
- 1/4 cup balsamic vinegar
- 2 tablespoons Dijon mustard
- 1 tablespoon honey
- Salt and pepper to taste
- 1/4 cup chopped fresh parsley

Instructions:

1. Preheat oven to 400°F (200°C).

2. In a medium saucepan, bring the quinoa and water to a boil.

3. Reduce the heat to low and simmer for 15-20 minutes or until the quinoa is tender.

4. Meanwhile, spread the mixed vegetables on a baking sheet and drizzle with the olive oil.

5. Roast the vegetables for 15-20 minutes or until tender and slightly browned.

6. In a small bowl, whisk together the balsamic vinegar, Dijon mustard, honey, salt and pepper to make the vinaigrette. 7. In a large bowl, combine the cooked quinoa, roasted vegetables,

and chopped parsley.

8. Drizzle the balsamic vinaigrette over the salad and toss to coat.

9. Serve the salad at room temperature or chilled.

Nutritional Information:

- Calories: 320
- Protein: 9g
- Fat: 11g
- Carbohydrates: 49g
- Fiber: 8g

Snacks

Roasted Chickpeas

Description of the Meal: Roasted chickpeas are a savory and satisfying snack that can be enjoyed anytime of the day. They are crispy on the outside and tender on the inside, with a delicious nutty flavor that pairs perfectly with a variety of spices.

Ingredients:

- 1 can of chickpeas, drained and rinsed
- 1 tablespoon olive oil
- 1 teaspoon smoked paprika
- 1 teaspoon garlic powder
- Salt and black pepper to taste

Instructions:

1. Preheat your oven to 400°F (200°C).

2. Pat the chickpeas dry with a paper towel.

3. In a mixing bowl, toss the chickpeas with olive oil, smoked paprika, garlic powder, salt, and black pepper until evenly coated.

4. Spread the chickpeas in a single layer on a baking sheet lined with parchment paper.

5. Roast the chickpeas for 20-25 minutes, or until crispy and golden brown.

6. Remove from the oven and let them cool for a few minutes before serving.

Nutritional Information:

- Calories: 124 kcal
- Protein: 5.6 g
- Fat: 4.1 g
- Carbohydrates: 16.4 g
- Fiber: 4.4 g

Greek Yogurt with Berries

Description of the Meal: Greek yogurt with berries is a delicious and healthy breakfast or snack option that is easy to make and packed with protein and antioxidants. The tangy flavor of the yogurt complements the sweetness of the berries, making it a satisfying and flavorful meal.

Ingredients:

- 1 cup of Greek yogurt
- 1/2 cup of mixed berries (strawberries, blueberries, raspberries)

- 1 tablespoon honey
- 1/4 teaspoon vanilla extract

Instructions:

1. In a bowl, mix the Greek yogurt, honey, and vanilla extract until well combined.

2. Wash and chop the berries.

3. Serve the yogurt in a bowl and top with the mixed berries.

Nutritional Information:

- Calories: 189 kcal
- Protein: 20.5 g
- Fat: 2.7 g
- Carbohydrates: 21.3 g
- Fiber: 2.2 g

Spicy Edamame

Description of the Meal: Spicy edamame is a popular Japanese appetizer that is easy to make and packed with protein and fiber. The edamame beans are steamed and then tossed with a spicy sauce, making it a healthy and flavorful snack.

Ingredients:

- 1 cup of edamame beans, shelled
- 1 tablespoon soy sauce
- 1 teaspoon sesame oil
- 1/4 teaspoon red pepper flakes
- 1/4 teaspoon garlic powder

Instructions:

1. Steam the shelled edamame beans for 5-7 minutes or until tender.

2. In a mixing bowl, combine soy sauce, sesame oil, red pepper flakes, and garlic powder.

3. Add the steamed edamame beans to the mixing bowl and toss until evenly coated with the spicy sauce.

4. Serve in a bowl and enjoy.

Nutritional Information:

- Calories: 121 kcal
- Protein: 10.2 g
- Fat: 5.8 g
- Carbohydrates: 10.5 g
- Fiber: 5.2 g

Hummus and Veggies

Description of the Meal: Hummus and veggies is a healthy and satisfying snack that is easy to make and perfect for dipping. The creamy texture of the hummus pairs well with the crispiness of the veggies, making it a delicious and nutritious snack.

Ingredients:

- 1 cup of hummus
- 1 cup of mixed veggies (carrots, celery, cucumber, bell pepper)
- Salt and black pepper to taste

Instructions:

1. Wash and chop the mixed veggies into bite-sized pieces.

2. Serve the hummus in a bowl and sprinkle salt and black pepper to taste.

3. Arrange the mixed veggies around the hummus bowl.

4. Use the veggies to scoop up the hummus and enjoy.

Nutritional Information:

- Calories: 148 kcal
- Protein: 6.1 g
- Fat: 9.6 g
- Carbohydrates: 12.2 g
- Fiber: 4.8 g

Trail Mix

Description of the Meal: Trail mix is a classic snack that is perfect for on-the-go or as a quick and easy snack at home. The combination of nuts, seeds, and dried fruits provides a variety of flavors and textures that are both satisfying and nutritious.

Ingredients:

- 1/2 cup of almonds
- 1/2 cup of cashews
- 1/2 cup of pumpkin seeds
- 1/2 cup of dried cranberries
- 1/4 cup of dark chocolate chips

Instructions:

1. In a mixing bowl, combine the almonds, cashews, pumpkin seeds, dried cranberries, and dark chocolate chips.

2. Mix the ingredients together until evenly distributed.

3. Serve in a bowl or divide into individual portions for on-the-go snacking.

Nutritional Information:

- Calories: 413 kcal
- Protein: 12.3 g
- Fat: 29.5 g
- Carbohydrates: 31.6 g
- Fiber: 5.9 g

Baked Sweet Potato Chips

Description of the Meal: Baked sweet potato chips are a healthy and delicious alternative to traditional potato chips. The sweet flavor of the sweet potatoes pairs well with a variety of seasonings, making it a versatile snack option.

Ingredients:

- 2 medium-sized sweet potatoes
- 2 tablespoons olive oil
- Salt and black pepper to taste

Instructions:

1. Preheat your oven to 375°F (190°C).

2. Wash and slice the sweet potatoes into thin rounds.

3. In a mixing bowl, toss the sweet potato slices with olive oil, salt, and black pepper until evenly coated.

4. Spread the sweet potato slices in a single layer on a

baking sheet lined with parchment paper.

5. Bake for 15-20 minutes or until golden brown and crispy.

6. Remove from the oven and let them cool for a few minutes before serving.

Nutritional Information:

- Calories: 132 kcal
- Protein: 1.5 g
- Fat: 6.3 g
- Carbohydrates: 18.1 g
- Fiber: 2.5 g

Almond Butter and Apple Slices

Description of the Meal: Almond butter and apple slices are a delicious and healthy snack that is perfect for satisfying your sweet tooth. The creamy texture of the almond butter pairs well with the crispiness of the apples, making it a satisfying and nutritious snack.

Ingredients:

- 2 medium-sized apples
- 2 tablespoons almond butter

Instructions:

1. Wash and slice the apples into thin rounds.

2. Spread almond butter on each apple slice.

3. Serve

Desserts

Greek Yogurt with Berries

Description of the Meal: Greek Yogurt with Berries is a healthy and delicious breakfast option that is perfect for starting your day. This meal is packed with protein, vitamins, and antioxidants, and it's a great way to fuel your body for the day ahead.

Ingredients:

- 1 cup of Greek yogurt
- 1/2 cup of mixed berries (strawberries, blueberries, and raspberries)
- 1 tablespoon of honey
- 1/4 cup of granola (optional)

Instructions:

1. In a bowl, mix the Greek yogurt and honey together.
2. Add the mixed berries on top of the yogurt.
3. Sprinkle granola on top, if desired.
4. Enjoy!

Nutritional Information: This meal provides approximately 250-300 calories, 20 grams of protein, and 10 grams of fiber.

Baked Pears with Walnuts

Description of the Meal: Baked Pears with Walnuts is a healthy and delicious dessert that is perfect for any occasion. This meal is rich in fiber, antioxidants, and healthy fats, making it a great choice for those who want to indulge in a sweet treat without the guilt.

Ingredients:

- 2 ripe pears

- 1/4 cup of chopped walnuts
- 1 tablespoon of honey
- 1/2 teaspoon of cinnamon

Instructions:

1. Preheat the oven to 375°F.
2. Cut the pears in half and remove the core.
3. Place the pears on a baking sheet.
4. In a small bowl, mix the chopped walnuts, honey, and cinnamon together.
5. Spoon the mixture over the pears.
6. Bake for 20-25 minutes, or until the pears are tender.
7. Enjoy!

Nutritional Information: This meal provides approximately 200-250 calories, 5 grams of protein, and 6 grams of fiber.

Chocolate Chia Seed Pudding

Description of the Meal: Chocolate Chia Seed Pudding is a healthy and delicious dessert that is perfect for satisfying your sweet tooth. This meal is packed with fiber, healthy fats, and antioxidants, making it a great choice for those who want to indulge in a dessert without the guilt.

Ingredients:

- 1/4 cup of chia seeds
- 1 cup of almond milk
- 1 tablespoon of cocoa powder
- 1 tablespoon of honey

- 1/2 teaspoon of vanilla extract

Instructions:

1. In a bowl, mix the chia seeds, almond milk, cocoa powder, honey, and vanilla extract together.

2. Cover the bowl with plastic wrap and refrigerate overnight.

3. In the morning, give the pudding a stir and add additional almond milk if desired.

4. Enjoy!

Nutritional Information: This meal provides approximately 250-300 calories, 8 grams of protein, and 10 grams of fiber.

Banana Oatmeal Cookies

Description of the Meal: Banana Oatmeal Cookies are a healthy and delicious snack that is perfect for any time of the day. These cookies are made with wholesome ingredients, and they're a great way to satisfy your sweet tooth without indulging in processed foods.

Ingredients:

- 2 ripe bananas
- 1 cup of rolled oats
- 1/4 cup of raisins
- 1/4 cup of chopped walnuts
- 1/4 cup of honey
- 1/2 teaspoon of cinnamon

Instructions:

1. Preheat the oven to 350°F.

2. In a bowl, mash the ripe bananas until smooth. 3. Add the rolled oats, raisins, chopped walnuts, honey, and cinnamon to the bowl, and mix until well combined.

4. Drop spoonfuls of the mixture onto a baking sheet lined with parchment paper.

5. Bake for 15-20 minutes, or until the cookies are golden brown.

6. Enjoy!

Nutritional Information: This meal provides approximately 100-150 calories per cookie, 2 grams of protein, and 3 grams of fiber.

Fruit Salad with Honey-Lemon Dressing

Description of the Meal: Fruit Salad with Honey-Lemon Dressing is a refreshing and healthy side dish that is perfect for any meal. This salad is packed with vitamins, antioxidants, and fiber, making it a great way to add more nutrition to your diet.

Ingredients:

- 2 cups of mixed fruit (pineapple, grapes, strawberries, and kiwi)
- 1 tablespoon of honey
- 1 tablespoon of lemon juice
- 1/2 teaspoon of vanilla extract

Instructions:

1. Wash and cut the fruit into bite-sized pieces.

2. In a small bowl, mix the honey, lemon juice, and vanilla extract together to make the dressing.

3. Pour the dressing over the fruit and toss to coat.

4. Chill in the refrigerator for at least 30 minutes.

5. Enjoy!

Nutritional Information: This meal provides approximately 100-150 calories, 1 gram of protein, and 3 grams of fiber per serving.

Vegan Avocado Chocolate Mousse

Description of the Meal: Vegan Avocado Chocolate Mousse is a healthy and decadent dessert that is perfect for satisfying your sweet tooth. This dessert is made with wholesome ingredients, and it's a great way to indulge in a treat without the guilt.

Ingredients:

- 2 ripe avocados
- 1/4 cup of cocoa powder
- 1/4 cup of maple syrup
- 1 teaspoon of vanilla extract
- 1/4 cup of almond milk

Instructions:

1. Cut the avocados in half, remove the pit, and scoop the flesh into a blender or food processor.

2. Add the cocoa powder, maple syrup, vanilla extract, and almond milk to the blender, and blend until smooth and creamy.

3. Chill in the refrigerator for at least 30 minutes.

4. Enjoy!

Nutritional Information: This meal provides approximately 200-250 calories, 3 grams of protein, and 5 grams of fiber per serving.

CHAPTER SIX

Explanation Of The Benefits Of Exercise

Exercise is an essential aspect of leading a healthy and active lifestyle. It is the physical activity that we undertake to maintain and improve our physical and mental health. There are numerous benefits of exercise, ranging from physical fitness, weight management, improved immunity, better sleep, and reduced risk of chronic diseases.

One of the significant benefits of exercise is that it helps in maintaining a healthy weight. Regular physical activity helps in burning calories and maintaining a healthy balance between the calories consumed and the calories burned. Exercise also helps in building lean muscle mass, which in turn helps in increasing the metabolic rate and burning more calories.

Exercise is also known to reduce the risk of chronic diseases such as cardiovascular disease, diabetes, and obesity. Physical activity helps in improving the cardiovascular system by reducing the levels of bad cholesterol and improving the circulation of blood in the body. It also helps in reducing the risk of type 2 diabetes by improving insulin sensitivity and blood sugar control.

Exercise also plays a crucial role in improving mental health and reducing stress levels. Physical activity helps in the release of endorphins, which are the feel-good hormones, thereby improving mood and reducing stress levels. Exercise also helps in improving cognitive function and reducing the risk of age-related cognitive decline.

Regular exercise also helps in improving sleep quality and reducing the risk of sleep disorders. It helps in promoting a healthy sleep pattern by improving the circadian rhythm and reducing the time taken to fall asleep.

In summary, exercise is essential for maintaining a healthy and active lifestyle. It helps in maintaining a healthy weight, reducing the risk of chronic diseases, improving mental health, and promoting better sleep quality.

Recommended Types Of Exercise

There are various types of exercises that can be undertaken to maintain physical fitness and improve overall health. It is recommended to undertake a combination of aerobic and strength training exercises for optimal health benefits.

Aerobic exercise is also known as cardiovascular exercise, and it involves activities that increase the heart and respiratory rates. Some examples of aerobic exercises include walking, jogging, swimming, cycling, and dancing. These exercises help in improving cardiovascular fitness, burning calories, and reducing the risk of chronic diseases.

Strength training exercises, also known as resistance training, involve activities that help in building lean muscle mass. These exercises include weightlifting, push-ups, squats, lunges, and pull-ups. Strength training exercises help in improving bone density, increasing metabolic rate, and improving overall physical function.

Flexibility and balance exercises are also essential for overall physical fitness. These exercises include stretching, yoga, and tai chi. These exercises help in improving flexibility, reducing the risk of falls, and promoting relaxation and stress reduction.

It is essential to consult a fitness professional or a physician before starting any exercise regimen, especially if you have any pre-existing medical conditions.

Tips For Incorporating Exercise Into Your Daily Routine

Incorporating exercise into your daily routine is crucial for maintaining an active and healthy lifestyle. Here are some tips for incorporating exercise into your daily routine:

1. Set realistic goals: Setting realistic goals is important for staying motivated and achieving your fitness objectives. Start small, and gradually increase the intensity and duration of your exercise routine.

2. Schedule exercise into your daily routine: Schedule exercise into your daily routine, just like any other appointment. This will help you prioritize exercise and ensure that you make time for it.

3. Find an exercise partner: Having an exercise partner can help in staying motivated and making exercise more fun. It also helps in holding each other accountable and sticking to a regular exercise routine.

4. Incorporate exercise into your daily activities:

Incorporate exercise into your daily activities, such as taking the stairs instead of the elevator, cycling to work, or taking a brisk walk during lunch breaks.

5. Choose activities that you enjoy: Choosing activities that you enjoy is crucial for maintaining a regular exercise routine. If you enjoy dancing, sign up for a dance class. If you love swimming, join a local swimming club. The key is to find activities that you enjoy and look forward to.

6. Mix up your exercise routine: Mixing up your exercise routine can help in preventing boredom and ensuring that you are working different muscle groups. Try different types of exercise, such as swimming, running, cycling, or yoga.

7. Use technology: Use technology to track your progress and stay motivated. There are various fitness apps and wearable devices that can help in tracking your fitness goals and progress.

8. Be patient and consistent: Consistency is key when it comes to exercise. It takes time and effort to see results, so be patient and consistent with your exercise routine.

In conclusion, incorporating exercise into your daily routine is essential for maintaining a healthy and active lifestyle. Setting realistic goals, scheduling exercise into your daily routine, finding an exercise partner, incorporating exercise into your daily activities, choosing activities that you enjoy, mixing up your exercise routine, using technology, and being patient and consistent are some tips for incorporating exercise into your daily routine.

CONCLUSION

Recap Of The Benefits Of The Blue Zone Diet Program

The Blue Zone Diet is a lifestyle-based eating plan that is designed to increase the lifespan and health of individuals by promoting healthy food choices and practices. It is based on the diet of individuals living in the Blue Zones, which are regions in the world that are known for their longevity and low rates of chronic diseases.

There are several benefits associated with following the Blue Zone Diet program:

1. Promotes a Plant-Based Diet

One of the key principles of the Blue Zone Diet is to consume a predominantly plant-based diet. This means that individuals are encouraged to consume vegetables, fruits, legumes, nuts, and whole grains, while minimizing their consumption of meat and processed foods. A plant-based diet is associated with numerous health benefits, such as reducing the risk of heart disease, stroke, and cancer.

2. Emphasizes Whole Foods

The Blue Zone Diet promotes the consumption of whole, minimally processed foods. Whole foods are nutrient-dense and are rich in fiber, vitamins, and minerals, which are essential for maintaining optimal health. By choosing whole foods over processed foods, individuals can reduce their intake of added sugars, unhealthy fats, and sodium, which are associated with an increased risk of chronic diseases.

3. Encourages Intermittent Fasting

Intermittent fasting is a practice that involves restricting the timing of food intake. The Blue Zone Diet encourages individuals to practice intermittent fasting by consuming their meals within a specific window of time, such as an 8-hour period. Intermittent fasting has been shown to improve metabolic health, reduce inflammation, and promote weight loss.

4. Supports Social Connections

The Blue Zone Diet emphasizes the importance of social connections and relationships. Eating meals with family and friends, joining social clubs or groups, and participating in community events are all encouraged. Social connections have been shown to improve mental health, reduce stress, and increase life expectancy.

5. Promotes Physical Activity

The Blue Zone Diet program encourages individuals to engage in regular physical activity, such as walking, biking, or swimming. Physical activity has numerous health benefits, such as reducing the risk of heart disease, stroke, and obesity. It also helps to improve mental health, reduce stress, and increase overall well-being.

Encouragement to Continue the Program for Long-Term Health Benefits

While the Blue Zone Diet program can provide numerous health benefits, it is important to continue the program over the long-term to achieve optimal results. Here are some tips for maintaining the program:

1. Set Realistic Goals

When starting the Blue Zone Diet program, it is important to set realistic goals. Start with small changes, such as adding more vegetables to your meals or reducing your intake of processed foods. As you become more comfortable with the program, you can gradually make additional changes.

2. Track Your Progress

Tracking your progress can help to keep you motivated and on track. Keep a food journal to track your meals and note how you feel after eating certain foods. You can also track your physical activity and monitor your weight and measurements over time.

3. Find Support

Finding support can be helpful when following the Blue Zone Diet program. Joining a support group or finding a friend who is also following the program can help to keep you motivated and accountable. You can also find support online through social media groups or forums.

4. Be Flexible

It is important to be flexible when following the Blue Zone Diet program. There may be times when it is difficult to follow the program, such as when traveling or attending social events. In these situations, try to make the healthiest choices possible and get back on track as soon as possible.

5. Celebrate Your Success

Celebrating your successes can help to keep you motivated and engaged in the program. When you achieve a goal, such as reducing your intake of processed foods or increasing your physical activity, take the time to acknowledge and celebrate your success. This can help to reinforce positive behaviors and make the program more enjoyable.

6. Focus on the Benefits

Focusing on the benefits of the Blue Zone Diet program can help to keep you motivated over the long-term. Remind yourself of the numerous health benefits, such as reducing the risk of chronic diseases and increasing lifespan. Additionally, focus on the positive changes you have experienced, such as increased energy levels or improved mood.

7. Make It a Lifestyle

To achieve long-term success with the Blue Zone Diet program, it is important to make it a lifestyle. This means incorporating the principles of the program into your daily life and making them a part of your routine. This can help to ensure that the program becomes a sustainable and enjoyable way of life.

8. Seek Professional Guidance

If you are unsure about how to follow the Blue Zone Diet program or have specific health concerns, consider seeking professional guidance. Registered dietitians and healthcare providers can provide personalized recommendations and support to help you achieve optimal results.

9. Stay Consistent

Consistency is key when following the Blue Zone Diet program. To achieve optimal results, it is important to consistently follow the principles of the program over the long-term. This can help to ensure that you achieve the numerous health benefits associated with the program.

www.ingramcontent.com/pod-product-compliance
Lightning Source LLC
Chambersburg PA
CBHW050656250726

48662CB00002B/707